A CLINICAL GUIDE TO THE MENOPAUSE AND THE POSTMENOPAUSE

A CLINICAL GUIDE TO

The Menopause

AND THE

Postmenopause

AYERST LABORATORIES

NEW YORK · MONTREAL

Published by Information Publishing Co., Inc.,
3 West 57th Street, New York City

Library of Congress catalog 68-57411

Contents

Management of Vaginal Bleeding
Management of Side Effects

Introduction

THE CLOSING YEARS of the female reproductive phase present the clinician with a particularly challenging complex of symptoms. During the course of this climacteric process, he is confronted with adverse effects that vary widely in intensity, and in time and order of appearance. Symptoms may persist over a brief span of months or for as long as a dozen years. Regardless of such variances, however, the physical and emotional consequences of the climacteric are frequently highly distressing and sometimes even disabling. They pose special problems of diagnosis and management.

When the female endocrine system was less well understood, far less could be done to ameliorate the symptoms associated with this time of waning ovarian function and dwindling estrogen output. Today, new concepts stemming from further investigations into hormonal mechanisms (discussed in this book) have made possible more effective management of the climacteric.

Although the terms *menopause* and *climacteric* are often used interchangeably, *menopause* more accurately describes the final menstrual period, *climacteric* the entire interval of the gradual transition from fertility and "femininity" to senescence and "old age." Ovarian production of estrogen begins to falter several years before the cessation of menstruation, and with this hormonal decline come symptoms that change in type because of the progressive nature of the process.

7

The premenopausal and menopausal years are marked by such classic signs as menstrual irregularity, hot flushes, sweats, irritability, and insomnia. The postmenopausal period often sees the female physiology achieving a gradual adjustment to hormonal decline and an abatement of these complaints. Frequently, however, the postmenopausal woman is afflicted with a new array of distressing symptoms, and with degenerative physiologic changes. Reproductive organs atrophy and the skin tends to lose turgor and to fall into wrinkles. In many women, decalcification of the bones results in loss of height and development of the "dowager's hump" of osteoporosis.

It is evident, then, that women are beset by—and clinicians confronted with—a variety of complaints over an extended interval—premenopausal, menopausal, and postmenopausal. Moreover, debilitating physiologic effects are intertwined with emotional problems—as the woman begins to appear and feel "old," she often tends toward a negative and depressed outlook on life.

The dimensions of this problem can be seen in the fact that menopause is occurring in American women today at a median age of forty-nine years. Since the modern woman's life expectancy is approximately seventy-five years, roughly one third of her existence may be marred by moderate to severe symptoms and sequelae of the climacteric. While some individuals remain asymptomatic except for changes in menstrual pattern, many millions of American women in their forties are at risk of developing distressing menopausal symptoms.

At the same time, a growing number of physicians no longer feel that the adverse consequences of the climacteric are inevitable and irreversible. More and more are regarding the process as an estrogen deficiency state that can be managed, as are other endocrine insufficiencies. They are utilizing estrogen replacement therapy not only to ameliorate climacteric-associated symptoms, but in efforts to retard such aging processes as organ and tissue atrophy, osteoporosis, and, possibly, atherosclerosis.

This brief publication will recapitulate current understanding of the climacteric, review the status of estrogen replacement therapy, and outline widely accepted procedures of diagnosis and patient management. Documentation is provided throughout for clinicians who may wish to consult full details in the literature. (SEE BIBLIOGRAPHY.)

First, the key role played by estrogen in the phases of a woman's life is summarized.

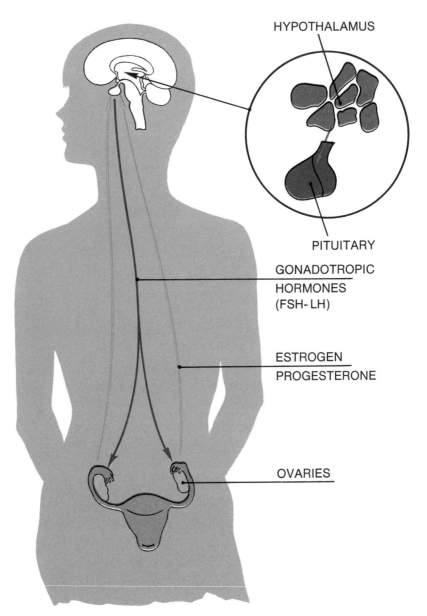

HYPOTHALAMUS

PITUITARY

GONADOTROPIC
HORMONES
(FSH- LH)

ESTROGEN
PROGESTERONE

OVARIES

FIG. 1   Diagram illustrates gonadotropic stimulation of ovaries to produce estrogen and progesterone; subsequent "feedback" inhibition of
hypothalamus and pituitary by these hormones is shown in enlarged
detail.

I

The Three Phases
of Woman

THE LIFE OF a woman can be divided into three major phases marked by the growth, activity, and involution of her reproductive organs. The changing endocrine interactions that characterize each phase have been described in great detail.[1-8]

GROWTH STAGE

Infancy through puberty

Although the pituitary and the ovaries make up the key organs of the female reproductive system, they do not become fully operational as a "femininity factor" until puberty has been completed. This endocrinologic relationship does not achieve maturity until adolescence, but the ovaries contain, at the time of birth, the primordial germ cells from which all ova subsequently develop. The number of these potential follicles in the ovaries at birth is estimated to be several hundred thousand; only about four hundred, however, will ever reach maturity.

Despite minimal ovarian function, small amounts of estrogen are evidently secreted in childhood; traces are excreted in the urine during this stage. Though insufficient for genital stimulation, early estrogen production is believed to influence the more rapid skeletal maturation and the earlier onset of puberty in the female.

During childhood, the hormones secreted by the anterior lobe of the pituitary chiefly influence metabolic functions and promote somatic growth and development. The pituitary then initiates the onset of puberty; the hypothalamus begins to stimulate the pituitary to produce gonadotropic hormones in preparation for gonadal development and the reproductive function. The pituitary begins to secrete follicle-stimulating hormone (FSH), and maturing ovarian follicles start to produce somewhat higher levels of estrogen; the FSH levels are not high enough, however, to evoke ovulation.

The first overt evidence that a pituitary-ovarian axis is functioning usually appears between the ages of 8 and 12. The higher levels of circulating estrogen cause the following physical changes to occur in sequence: broadening of the pelvis, budding of the nipples and breasts, development of the vaginal mucosa, growth of the external and internal genitalia, pigmentation of the nipples, enlargement of the breasts, and menarche. Estrogen also stimulates skeletal maturation and the deposition of fat to round out body contours.

The first menstrual flow usually appears between the twelfth and fifteenth year, the average age being thirteen and a half years. The bleeding involved in menarche usually is not true menstruation since it occurs in most cases without ovulation. Two years generally elapse before anovulatory bleeding gives way to regular ovulation and true menstruation.

ACTIVITY STAGE

Childbearing years

In the mature woman, the biologic object of femaleness—pregnancy—is anticipated in the endometrium, via a dynamic interplay between the pituitary and ovarian hormones. The following description presents the basic concept of this coordinated and interdependent hormonal interaction. (FIG. 1.)

Gonadotropic hormones (gonadotropins, affecting the ovaries) are secreted by the pituitary under hypothalamic stimulation and, in turn, stimulate the secretion of ovarian hormones. In relation to each normal menstrual cycle, five hormones are elaborated.

PITUITARY	OVARIES
follicle-stimulating hormone (FSH)	estrogen
luteinizing hormone (LH)	progesterone
luteotropic hormone (Lut H)	

Through a "feedback" mechanism, the ovarian "female sex hormones" exert an inhibitory effect on the pituitary when they reach high concentrations. High levels of estrogen and progesterone first reduce and then block pituitary production of the three gonadotropic hormones.

This ebb and flow of hormonal influences and counterinfluences lies at the heart of the changes that characterize the normal menstrual cycle.

As FIG. 2 shows, both the pituitary-ovarian interactions and the endometrial responses are determined by the circulating levels of estrogen and progesterone.

13

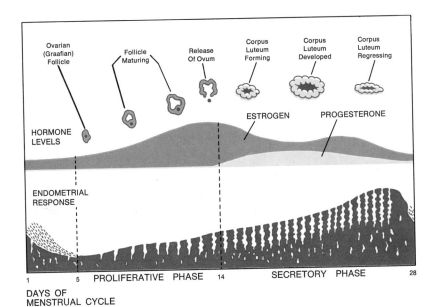

FIG. 2 Development of ovarian follicle, production of ovarian hormones, and changes in endometrium during menstrual cycle.

Menstrual cycle

Days 1 through 14   The first half of the menstrual cycle (referred to variously as the preovulatory, follicular, and proliferative phase) is characterized by marked proliferation of the endometrium. This occurs because estrogen, whose levels have been rising, is essentially a "growth" hormone to the endometrium.

Under the predominating stimulus of FSH, several ovarian (or graafian) follicles, each containing an ovum, begin to develop. A small amount of LH is believed to complement FSH in promoting the anatomical development of the follicles during this preovulatory phase, and to be necessary to their functional or secretory activity. Usually only one follicle achieves maturity, while the others gradually undergo atresia.

14

At midcycle, under the continuing stimulation of FSH and the strongly increasing influence of LH, the mature graafian follicle ruptures, releasing the ovum. The high estrogen content of the follicular fluid then increases the circulating estrogen to levels which begin to inhibit the pituitary secretion of FSH. However, the secretion of luteinizing hormone continues.

Days 15 through 28   After the ovum has been expelled, the ruptured follicle is converted into a corpus luteum under the influence of persistent LH secretion. With the additional influence of the luteotropic hormone (Lut H) from the pituitary, the corpus luteum is activated to secrete both estrogen and progesterone, the "pregnancy hormone," or the hormone of potential or actual pregnancy.

During the second half of the menstrual cycle (the progestational, luteal, or secretory phase), the proliferative endometrium is converted into the secretory type capable of receiving and nourishing a fertilized ovum. This change occurs in response to the elaboration of progesterone in addition to estrogen.

The average functional life of a corpus luteum—the period during which it manufactures progesterone and estrogen—is twelve to fourteen days, unless its life is prolonged by pregnancy. During peak activity (about midpoint in the second half of the cycle), it produces high levels of estrogen and progesterone, which in turn act to inhibit the pituitary elaboration of LH and Lut H. This inhibition is followed by regression of the corpus luteum in the terminal part of the cycle. Eventual involution of the corpus brings about a sharp reduction in estrogen levels and, essentially, the disappearance of progesterone.

Menstruation is preceded by a marked decrease in estrogen and progesterone levels, usually occurring about 24 hours before endometrial regression. True menstrual bleeding follows within a few days, and normally continues until the endometrium has been reduced to its basal layers. (As FIG. 2 shows, the next menstrual cycle is considered to begin with the first day of bleeding.)

15

INVOLUTION STAGE

The climacteric

The process of aging brings about progressive and irreversible changes in the ovaries, leading to the loss of childbearing capability. The primordial follicles which had been abundant become depleted with time, and their ability to mature declines; finally, ovulation ceases. As a consequence, cyclic production of progesterone fails to occur and estrogen levels fall below the amount necessary to induce endometrial bleeding. Menstruation becomes irregular, more widely spaced, and eventually ceases; total cessation marks the occurrence of the menopause.

The pituitary remains functional, but in effect the aging ovary becomes increasingly incapable of responding to its stimulation. In turn, the pituitary, no longer under the normal cyclic influence of ovarian hormones, becomes hyperactive, producing excessive amounts of gonadotropins.

The end result of this decline in ovarian function is a disturbance of endocrine balance, and it is to this imbalance that many distressing symptoms of the climacteric appear to be related. In the following section, some of the more commonly encountered climacteric symptoms are described in detail.

II

The Climacteric: Changes and Symptoms

As ESTROGEN PRODUCTION ebbs during the climacteric years, many alterations in the body's structures and metabolism occur. These changes give rise to a multiplicity of symptoms and subjective complaints, some of which are suffered to some degree by an estimated eighty per cent of menopausal women.[6] A considerable number of these phenomena have been related directly to declining estrogen levels. Some may result from aging processes which are accelerated by estrogen insufficiency, while still others appear to be influenced or exacerbated by emotional and psychosomatic factors.

Wide variations have been seen in the severity of climacteric manifestations, and in the time of their appearance. Some women remain free of symptoms except for the irregular menses that usually precede menopause; the hormonal and physical changes evidently proceed so gradually that the effects are imperceptible to such persons. At the opposite extreme, women who undergo premature menopause as a result of castration, irradiation, or certain diseases are likely to experience severe symptoms and rapid degenerative changes due to sudden and complete loss of ovarian

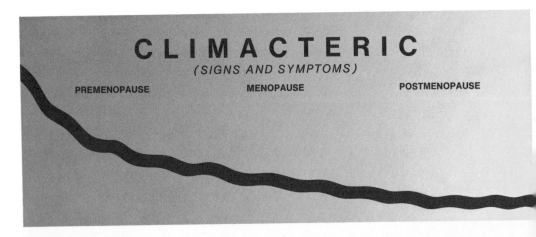

CLIMACTERIC
(SIGNS AND SYMPTOMS)

PREMENOPAUSE   **MENOPAUSE**   **POSTMENOPAUSE**

Menstrual irregularities	Cessation of menstruation	Senile vaginitis and pruritus vulvae
Early manifestations of vasomotor disturbances — *i.e.,* hot flushes, sweats, palpitations	Frequent manifestations of vasomotor disturbances	Occasional manifestations of vasomotor disturbances
Nervous symptoms — *i.e.,* excitability, irritability, insomnia, headache	Incipient atrophy of genitourinary tissues and structures related to loss of estrogen	Atrophy of urogenital structures leading to uterine prolapse, rectocele, cystocele
	"Silent" onset of bone resorption with related low back pain	Progressive bone resorption leading to osteoporosis and loss of height
	Generally negative outlook on life	

Fig. 3   Symptoms occurring with decline of estrogen. Both time of onset and rate of decline vary with individuals; symptoms may overlap between climacteric phases.

function.[9] Such an abrupt decline of estrogen levels usually precipitates a greater degree of hormonal imbalance and more severe reactions, particularly in women with a predisposing emotional instability.

Most women, however, follow no set pattern. Their climacteric signs and symptoms may begin well before the cessation of menstruation, appear at approximately the same time as menopause, or may not develop until years after menses have stopped. (FIG. 3.)

MENSTRUAL DISTURBANCES

The first overt sign of the climacteric is frequently observed as a change in the menstrual pattern. As ovulation and the production of progesterone cease, bleeding occurs from a proliferative endometrium, and the cycle may consequently be shortened by as much as a week. As ovarian function declines further, the cycle may become lengthened, since estrogen production is lower and a longer period of endometrial stimulation may be required to cause bleeding. The flow usually tapers off in quantity and duration. In some women cyclic bleeding is missed for a month, resumes, then is absent for longer intervals, and finally ceases after a two or three year period of irregularity. In a small minority, menstruation ceases abruptly.[2,3,8,10]

However, episodes of excessive bleeding are not uncommon before the menopause. Prolonged although not necessarily excessive estrogen production by persistent, unruptured ovarian follicles often results in endometrial hyperplasia, particularly the "Swiss-cheese" histologic type that is characterized by large, dilated mucosal glands. In the absence of progesterone, the hyperplastic endometrium may give rise to dysfunctional bleeding. However, any bleeding that is excessively profuse or prolonged, or that occurs intermenstrually, is considered to require careful investigation to rule out the presence of organic lesions, which increase in frequency among women of this age group.[3,11]

19

THE MENOPAUSAL SYNDROME

Subjective symptoms relating to almost every system of the body may develop around the time of the menopause, and are generally regarded as signs of the "menopausal syndrome."

Some signs even precede menopause. For example, the breasts may become turgid and tender and even increase in size, probably as a result of the unmodified effect of estrogen during anovulatory cycles and also, it is thought, because of increased pituitary stimulation. At this time cystic mastitis and other fibrocystic conditions of the breasts may develop or grow worse.[8]

Vasomotor symptoms

The most frequently reported features of the menopausal syndrome itself are hot flushes and sweats that result from vasomotor instability. Although the precise hormonal mechanism that produces these symptoms has not yet been identified, they are almost invariably relieved by estrogen therapy. The weight of etiologic evidence points to a disturbance in the equilibrium between the hypothalamus and the autonomic nervous system, both of which apparently become conditioned to a high estrogen level and then react to its decline.[12,13]

Typical hot flushes are experienced as sudden, wave-like sensations of heat that move up from the rib cage to envelop the chest, neck, and head, and are often accompanied by patchy erythemas of the skin. The flushes are frequently followed by profuse perspiration and terminate in a highly distressing feeling of chilliness. Attacks usually last from a few seconds to a half hour, but may persist for an hour, and even longer in some patients. They may occur once or twice a day, or as frequently as every half hour. They are especially disturbing at night, interfering with sleep; perspiration may be so drenching as to require a change of bedclothes.

Flushes and sweats are usually more severe in anxious women, and are intensified in most patients by excitement or stress.[8,14,15]

Symptoms with an emotional component

While the endocrine basis is unclear for many emotional manifestations and vague psychosomatic complaints that are considered part of the menopausal syndrome, there seems little doubt that the endocrine upheaval of menopause does influence these disturbances, sometimes by exaggerating the premenopausal emotional pattern.[16]

Emotional symptoms that are frequently mentioned include feelings of nervousness, irritability, depression, melancholia, hopelessness, and worthlessness, as well as weepiness, frigidity, impairment of memory, and difficulty in concentrating. Common subjective complaints are insomnia, vertigo, headache, tachycardia, palpitations, and fatigability. Some patients complain of muscle, joint, and backaches; vague abdominal pains, nausea and vomiting, flatulence, loss of appetite, constipation, and diarrhea; numbness and crawling sensations of the skin; "spots before the eyes" and "ringing in the ears," and sensations of choking and suffocation. Headaches, which approximately one third of menopausal patients cite as a new symptom, are usually of the "nervous tension" type, rarely migraine.[8,14,15,17-20]

These symptoms have often been considered to stem primarily from a psychological reaction, usually an expression of anxiety caused by the dramatic shifts in personal identity that confront some women during the climacteric. Many feel that in losing the ability to become pregnant, they are losing the essence of their femininity. Moreover, their children are grown or approaching adulthood and no longer need "mothering." Some fear the approach of old age, with its dreaded decline in attractiveness and libido, and many realize that their youthful hopes and aspirations

21

will never be fulfilled. These harsh adjustments pose a serious threat to the psychological foundation on which their ego structure is built.[16,21]

It has been noted that many patients who manifest severe psychological reactions during the climacteric have suffered earlier emotional problems which were only partially resolved during the years of reproductive maturity.

But some patients who develop intense emotional symptoms have previously been considered well adjusted—even noted as "active good citizens" in their communities. If their self-esteem had been based primarily on such activities and on exemplary child rearing, their changing status and decreasing stamina at menopause may be perceived as disastrous. Their initial anxiety may be followed by a deep sense of grief, which sometimes progresses to a psychoneurotic depressive reaction. Eventually, personality reorganization takes place, either through constructive adaptation or through increasing frustration, which may, on occasion, develop slowly into involutional melancholia. In such cases, early psychotherapeutic intervention by the physician, largely of a supportive nature, may effectively treat depressive reactions and possibly prevent more serious involutional disorders.[16,22]

Since estrogen replacement therapy may also mitigate various emotional and psychosomatic manifestations of the climacteric, hormonal deficiency is considered to make some contribution to their etiology. A recent study[23] concludes that specific symptoms may be related to estrogen deficiency in some patients and not in others; therefore, a given symptom may be completely relieved in some patients and persist in others. A placebo explanation is thought unlikely since patient response is often selective, with several symptoms alleviated and others unimproved. Such common symptoms as depression, insomnia, and headache appear to the investigator to be related to insufficient estrogen in approximately half of patients presenting with the menopausal syndrome.[23]

ATROPHIC CONDITIONS

Research evidence points strongly to an estrogen deficiency as the cause of marked regressive changes that occur in many body structures during the climacteric. Atrophy affects the skin, mucous membranes, and all of the reproductive organs, and is particularly evident in the genitalia, where it gives rise to a spectrum of distressing symptoms.

The vagina gradually shortens and becomes narrower and less elastic. The vaginal mucosa progressively loses its cornified epithelium, and finally consists of ten or fewer cell layers. The vaginal smear reflects increasing estrogen deficiency as the number of superficial cells decreases, and the proportion of intermediate cells, and then parabasal cells, rises. [24,25]

These degenerative changes may progress to atrophic vaginitis early in the climacteric, but this occurs more commonly some years after menopause. Clinically, estrogen deficiency causes the vaginal mucosa to become pale from decreasing vascularity, as well as extremely fragile. Its surface is easily eroded, may bleed, become ulcerated, and develop adhesions. Estrogen deficiency also permits the normally acidic vaginal secretions to become alkaline or only slightly acidic, thus increasing susceptibility to infection, even by organisms of normally low virulence. Often seen is a profuse, purulent discharge that excoriates the vulva. Patients complain of increasing dyspareunia, and of irritation and severe pruritus vulvae.[14,25-27]

Only mild atrophic changes may occur in the external genitalia during the climacteric, but they often become marked during senescence. There is loss of subcutaneous fat and shrinkage of tissues and structures.[24,25]

Atrophic changes due to an estrogen deficiency also affect the pelvic organs. The supporting structures of the uterus, bladder, and rectum lose tone and strength, favoring the development of uterine prolapse, cystocele, and rectocele. The linings of the urethra and neck of the bladder undergo thinning similar to that occurring in the vaginal mucosa and become susceptible to irritation. Caruncles often develop at the urethral meatus. The bladder sphincter may also lose tone. These alterations often lead to such symptoms as urgency, frequency, pain on voiding, and incontinence.[12,25,28]

General symptoms

Widespread changes also occur in the integument with estrogen deprivation and aging. The skin as a whole becomes thinner and loses elasticity and turgor. There is less hydration in the subcuticular layer. Scaling and wrinkles gradually appear. Palms and soles may develop the hardened plaques of keratoderma climacterium, and the mucous membranes of the nose and paranasal sinuses often become dry, paving the way for atrophic rhinitis.[29-31]

After menopause, the breasts usually shrink and droop as fat, glandular tissue, and tone decrease. The nipples become smaller and lose their erectile character.[8,25]

METABOLIC CHANGES

Osteoporosis

In the decades following menopause, women show a much greater tendency than do men of comparable age to develop osteoporotic decalcification of the bones. Considerable study is now seeking to determine the relationship between the high incidence of this disorder in postmenopausal women and the long term metabolic effects of estrogen decline.[32-36] (FIG. 4.)

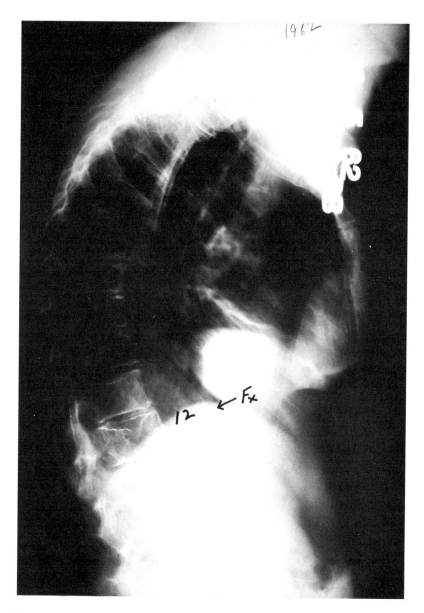

FIG. 4 Advanced osteoporosis revealed by lateral x-ray of spine of postmenopausal woman. Vertebrae show bone compression; note compression fracture of twelfth thoracic vertebra (arrow). Kyphosis, or "dowager's hump," is also evident.

A close association between estrogen deficiency and osteoporosis, which produces symptoms in approximately twenty-five per cent of postmenopausal women, is suggested by numerous studies. The findings show that osteoporosis develops earlier in women who undergo premature menopause as a result of castration. Estrogen therapy has long been accepted as the treatment of choice to relieve severe pain in the lower back, a frequent result of osteoporosis. While not reversing preexisting damage, it apparently helps to arrest further mineral loss from osteoporotic bones.[32-35,37,38]

Osteoporosis is not a single entity, but a nonspecific reaction of the skeleton to a variety of factors, including immobilization, hypogonadism, and an excess of catabolic hormones from the adrenal cortex or the thyroid. Furthermore, other disease states, such as myeloma, osteomalacia, and various arthropathies can mimic the subjective symptoms of osteoporosis and must be excluded by differential diagnosis.[33,38-40]

The most common first symptom of osteoporosis is a severe sudden backache, often following muscular effort or trauma, which lasts three or four weeks and may be interpreted as "lumbago." Eventually the backache becomes more or less chronic as increasing bone loss from the vertebrae causes compression fractures. An important early physical sign is loss of stature due to shortening of the trunk. The "dowager's hump" of older women is a familiar consequence of advanced postmenopausal osteoporosis, as is susceptibility to hip fractures. Roentgenographic evidence of bone demineralization usually cannot be obtained until the process is fairly well advanced—more than thirty per cent of calcium must be lost before increased radiolucency shows up clearly on conventional x-rays.[33,38,40]

The underlying disorder in osteoporosis is an inability of new bone formation to keep pace with bone resorption, the deficit manifesting itself in decreased density and increased porosity of the skeleton. A long-standing explanation of the postmenopausal form of the condition has held that estrogen deficiency deprives the osteoblasts of a necessary stimulus to the formation of bone matrix, around which calcium is deposited to form new bone tissue. A conflicting hypothesis has attributed osteoporosis to inadequate dietary intake of calcium and a consequent negative calcium balance. However, recent studies utilizing new technics for measuring bone density and mineral deposition indicate that estrogen exerts an anticatabolic effect on skeletal tissue, and thus prevents the excessive bone resorption that usually starts at menopause. This finding would not only account for the inability of estrogen replacement to restore lost bone, but could affirm its prophylactic value in most postmenopausal women.[32-34,36,39,41-43]

Atherosclerosis

Since premenopausal women show a relatively lower incidence of atherosclerosis which rises in the years following the menopause, the question of whether declining estrogen production is responsible for the striking rise in coronary heart disease in older women is under intensive investigation. Long-range studies have set out to determine whether estrogen therapy can extend the earlier relative immunity. Current evidence indicates that the relative incidence of coronary heart disease is at least 15 to 20 times greater in men than in women under the age of 40, but that the disparity recedes rapidly after the menopause. Manifestations of atherosclerosis also appear to be more common and severe among women who undergo premature menopause as a result of castration than among control group women of the same age, although this question is not thoroughly resolved.[12,44-47]

Clinical studies suggest a rise in serum cholesterol after the menopause; however, more long term investigations are needed to substantiate this phenomenon. Studies in process indicate that

27

the administration of estrogen alters this lipid pattern in the direction of lower total serum cholesterol, increased alpha-lipo-protein, and a lower cholesterol-phospholipid ratio—changes that are currently considered desirable in achieving primary and secondary prevention of atherosclerosis. One long term study of the effects of estrogen therapy in female castrates revealed fewer abnormal electrocardiograms than among untreated postmenopausal and castrated women.[44,48]

III

Diagnosis

ALTHOUGH ovarian steroid production virtually ceases with the menopause, a small but significant percentage of postmenopausal women show evidence of adequate estrogen production, presumably by the adrenal glands, throughout their remaining years.[9] In those who do not, a variety of diagnostic methods are used to verify the presence of estrogen deficiency.

Biochemical assay technics can measure estrogen levels precisely, but they are too costly for routine clinical use. Therefore, diagnosis is often based largely on the presence of such clear-cut menopausal symptoms as vasomotor phenomena and atrophic changes of the vagina. When symptoms are primarily subjective, a therapeutic trial with estrogen has been found helpful in establishing their relationship to hormonal insufficiency.[17,23,49]

Because the vaginal mucosa exhibits marked sensitivity to endogenous and exogenous estrogen, vaginal cytology has been considered a valuable guide to hormonal status. The smear is obtained from the lateral wall of the upper third of the vagina. Essentially the same staining technic recommended for Papani-

29

colaou smears may be followed. Recently developed rapid stains make it possible to prepare slides for viewing in less than a minute, if the physician wishes to have this done in his office. Or the smear may be inspected in a wet, unstained condition.[50-52]

The various types of cells seen in vaginal smears can be grouped according to several classification systems based on their cytoplasmic and nuclear characteristics. The least complex system divides them into three cytologic categories—superficial, intermediate, and parabasal cells. (More complicated systems refer to the superficial cells as "cornified," and place some of the intermediate cells in a fourth category called "precornified.")

Following the simplest system, adequate estrogen levels are indicated when a smear contains predominantly superficial cells. These are large, flattened cells containing small, deeply staining nuclei. Conversely, marked estrogen deficiency is reflected by the complete absence of superficial cells, and the presence of parabasal cells from the deeper layers of the vaginal epithelium. Intermediate cells are fairly large and flattened and contain large vesicular nuclei. Parabasal cells are small, round or oval, and contain very large vesicular nuclei.[51-53] (FIG. 5.)

Although vaginal smears have been the primary guide to the diagnosis and treatment of estrogen deficiency, it has been found that they do not always reflect true estrogen levels. The interplay of other hormones with estrogen, as well as such factors as vaginal infection, tissue sensitivity, and the effects of certain diseases and medications, may influence the clinical picture. Because of these complicating factors, smears from some young menstruating women fail to reflect the high estrogen levels they clearly possess. Similarly, smears from some postmenopausal patients do not reveal regressive cell changes despite undoubted estrogen deficiencies. Moreover, smear findings do not invariably correlate with menopausal symptoms or with a patient's response to therapy.[15,23,54]

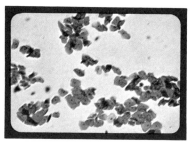

Normal 21-year-old woman. Approximately two-thirds of cells are large, pink-staining superficial, with small nuclei.

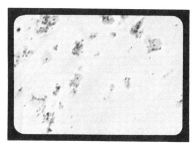

Estrogen-deficient menopausal woman, aged 47. Few superficial cells; majority are blue-staining intermediate and parabasal.

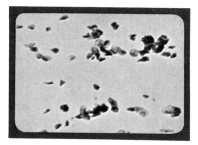

Same woman after estrogen therapy; approximately one-fourth of cells are now superficial.

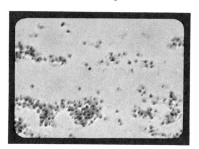

Estrogen-deficient postmenopausal woman, aged 61. Virtually all cells are blue-staining parabasal, with large nuclei.

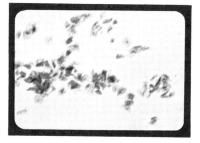

Same woman after estrogen treatment; approximately half the cells are now superficial, indicating excellent therapeutic response.

FIG. 5. Vaginal smears show typical cytologic variations: with adequate estrogen levels, with estrogen deficiency, and after estrogen replacement therapy.

Slides provided courtesy of T: J. Lin, M.D.

Since there are differing views of what constitutes a "normal" smear, particularly after the menopause, less clinical emphasis is currently being placed on strict interpretations of vaginal cytology. The procedure is considered to yield an approximate but still useful estimate of estrogen levels. And serial smears are especially helpful in evaluating the progression and regression of atrophic changes during prolonged observation of patients.[17,23,51]

DIFFERENTIAL DIAGNOSIS

Symptoms characteristic of the menopausal syndrome cannot be attributed to the climacteric purely on the basis of a patient's age. Some organic diseases are known to present symptoms similar to those of the menopausal syndrome, creating problems of differential diagnosis. Furthermore, signs of coexisting illnesses may at times be masked by severe menopausal symptoms.[28,55]

A detailed history, a thorough physical examination, and appropriate laboratory procedures provide valuable assistance in ruling out organic disorders that occur frequently during the climacteric years. These include diabetes, hypertension, and hyperthyroidism, as well as cardiovascular, renal, and gallbladder diseases. Careful interrogation and examination of a patient complaining of hot flushes may reveal that the symptoms never occur at night, and that they result from hypertension rather than the menopause. Similarly, radiologic and laboratory evaluation of a patient who suffers from severe night sweats may indicate the presence of tuberculosis.[17,28,55]

Early manifestations of the climacteric may be difficult to validate. Most physicians hesitate to make a diagnosis of menopausal syndrome when a patient is still having menstrual periods, especially if vasomotor symptoms are not prominent features of the clinical picture. When symptoms are suspected of being primarily psychogenic in origin, it is helpful to have a detailed history that includes data on the patient's emotional, marital, and family background. A psychosomatic component is considered to be more likely in individuals with a history of dysmenorrhea, infertility, and premenstrual tension. Marital difficulties have also been found to intensify climacteric symptoms. The role that emotional factors play in complaints depends to a large extent on a patient's previous psychic adaptation and her ability to accept the changes in social and psychological roles so common at this time of life.[14,16,55]

When amenorrhea first manifests itself during the climacteric, it frequently arouses fear of pregnancy in patients. A careful pelvic examination and demonstration of arborization in a dried sample of cervical mucus ordinarily rule out this possibility. Because of the increase in gonadotropin levels that occurs during the climacteric, biologic pregnancy tests often yield false positive results. Conversely, urinary gonadotropin assays are useful in establishing a diagnosis of early menopause, although a single test may be misleading. In most cases, such assays are unnecessary, and menopause is regarded to have occurred when menses have been absent for a full year.[11,14,28]

Pelvic findings are of utmost diagnostic importance during the climacteric. If there is a history of abnormal bleeding, curettage may be necessary to rule out uterine pathology. Breast examination is, of course, essential to ensure that mammary cancer is not present.[28]

Because of the high incidence of osteoporosis among women after menopause, it has been suggested that diagnostic workups include oblique or lateral radiographic films of the spine. These may reveal objective evidence of osteoporosis in the form of increased radiolucency or structural changes in the vertebrae. They also serve as a base line against which future loss in bone density may be measured.[40,56]

IV

Treatment

AN INCREASING NUMBER of investigators have been reporting on the efficacy of estrogen replacement therapy in the management of symptoms and sequelae associated with the menopause and the later years of the climacteric.[12-15,23,30,31,55,57-67] Inasmuch as most clinicians individualize treatment regimens to meet the needs of specific patients, therapeutic goals and approaches to the replacement of estrogen vary considerably, largely depending on the age, symptomatology, and history of patients. Despite this diversity, several main trends and approaches are gaining wide clinical acceptance.

GROWING APPLICATION OF ESTROGEN THERAPY

At one time, estrogen replacement therapy was reserved for patients suffering extreme manifestations of the menopause, particularly severe vasomotor flushes and sweats. Since these symp-

34

toms rarely last more than a year or two, estrogen therapy was gradually withdrawn. The primary aim of treatment was to ease the patient's physiologic adjustment to the declining estrogen levels of the menopausal period. Some clinicians continue to hold this view.[28,68]

However, the growing body of evidence that associates post-menopausal estrogen deficiency with the development of atrophic structural disorders, and an increased incidence of osteoporosis and atherosclerosis, has led many physicians to adopt a preventive approach to therapy.[12,15,49,57,61,67] Estrogen replacement is consequently being extended to more patients for longer periods.

In line with this preventive philosophy, the circumstances have broadened in which estrogen replacement treatment may be instituted. Several investigators consider that estrogenic therapy should be offered to essentially every postmenopausal woman.[57,61] Another concludes, "The menopausal woman must be considered a physiologic castrate, and replacement therapy should be administered to everyone with evidence of an estrogen lack."[12] As noted earlier, estrogen deficiency may be recognized by major alterations of the menstrual function, clear-cut symptoms of the menopausal syndrome, and gross or cytologic evidence of vaginal atrophy.

In older postmenopausal women, the development of dyspareunia, vulval degeneration, prolapse, bladder complaints, and osteoporosis are widely considered to be indications of a probable need for estrogen replacement.[55,67]

Efforts to prevent or retard climacteric phenomena are encouraging a trend toward long term estrogen therapy. A continued regimen in the postmenopausal or geriatric patient has been described as wise and appropriate therapy to retard the aging process.[17] Furthermore, many clinicians see no logical reason to discontinue replacement estrogen in a normal postmenopausal woman.[14,57]

Few conditions exist in which estrogen replacement therapy has been completely contraindicated. Traditionally, estrogen has been withheld from patients with a history of mammary or uterine cancer. However, some clinicians employ it when convinced that a malignant tumor has been eradicated. Since estrogen has a tendency to cause retention of salt and water, it is usually not prescribed for patients with severe kidney disease or cardiac decompensation. The advisability of administering estrogen to patients with a history of endometriosis or fibroids varies according to the case, but flare-ups have been found rare when the dosage is low. Untreated atypical endometrial hyperplasia and significant liver disease are two other conditions in which the hormone is often withheld.[12,13,49,61]

TYPES OF THERAPEUTIC REGIMENS

Orally administered estrogen is usually preferred inasmuch as it permits maintenance of more constant hormone levels than can be achieved with injectable forms of estrogen.

Local therapy in the form of an estrogenic cream, ointment, or suppository, is often used in the management of atrophic conditions of the vagina, vulva, and urethra. It brings prompt relief, but there is some difference of opinion whether local treatment alone is adequate for atrophic vaginitis. Oral therapy is being used increasingly in such cases because it is now thought that local evidence of estrogen deficiency indicates the probability that atrophic changes may be occurring throughout the body. Local and systemic therapy are frequently given simultaneously until urogenital symptoms have been controlled. Local preparations containing both estrogen and corticoids have been found particularly effective in relieving pruritus vulvae.[55,61]

When oral estrogen is indicated, some investigators[15,61,67] believe it should be taken in continuous daily doses; the majority of clinicians appear to prefer cyclic administration for three or four weeks followed by an interruption of one week.[12,13,30,50,58,64] Many factors are involved in the choice between these two types of therapy. The history, symptoms, and age of the patient are important, and dosage requirements may also influence the decision. But the most basic consideration is the inherent tendency of estrogen to cause tissue proliferation and uterine bleeding.

One reason for the wide adoption of a cyclic regimen is to provide for a regular interruption of tissue stimulation and thus avoid hypertrophy. Moreover, some investigators consider that fluctuating estrogen levels are such an integral part of female homeostasis that they insist on cyclic administration of estrogen even in hysterectomized patients.[13,68] Others believe that interrupting replacement therapy in postmenopausal patients is unnecessary, irrespective of whether they have intact uteri, and that interruption may result in the reappearance of symptoms during the intervals of nonmedication.[15,55,59,61,67]

Irregular bleeding is a common consequence of estrogen therapy in patients with intact uteri. Although, in general, smaller doses of estrogen are less likely to induce uterine bleeding, no therapeutic regimen can guarantee the prevention of this phenomenon.[8,28]

To control tendencies toward bleeding or hyperplasia, some clinicians consider it desirable to add progesterone to the estrogen replacement regimen.[50] Given for approximately five to ten days at the end of an estrogen therapy cycle, or at intervals during continuous therapy, progesterone promotes complete endometrial shedding in a predictable, self-limiting menstrual period. This "medical curettage" avoids protracted bleeding, which may occur with unopposed estrogen therapy. Opinions vary as to whether medical curettage should be employed regularly, in effect continuing the menstrual function well beyond the time of normal menopause, or infrequently, when there is a specific indication that endometrial shedding is advisable. No evidence has been advanced that progesterone plays a desirable role in the nonreproductive physiology of the body that should be continued after menopause.[15,28,58,69]

INDIVIDUALIZATION OF THERAPY

The climacteric patient should be encouraged to see her physician at least twice a year so therapy can be tailored to her individual needs. Since a rationale exists for many different regimens of estrogen replacement, many physicians consider it appropriate to try several dosage schedules, if necessary, to find the one most effective for a given patient. Therapy is usually started at an average dose, and increased if symptoms are not relieved. However, some clinicians prefer to start with a relatively large dose to bring symptoms under prompt control, and then taper the dosage.[8]

Some clinicians periodically reduce or suspend the administration of estrogen for a few weeks during treatment to determine whether it is still needed. Others have noted that older patients can often be switched from cyclic therapy to small maintenance doses given every two or three days on a continuous basis.[23] Patients who show signs of postmenopausal osteoporosis are usually maintained on a regimen that includes not only high dosage estrogen replacement, but also dietary supplements and regular exercise as adjunctive measures.[38,70,71]

Gynecologists recommend that the periodic checkup of patients receiving menopausal therapy include a thorough physical examination, palpation of the breasts, inspection of the cervix, and cytologic studies of the cervix and vagina. They point out that these follow-up visits also provide excellent opportunities for providing simple supportive psychotherapy in the form of factual explanations and reassurance. A foremost need of a patient suffering from menopausal anxiety is for a sympathetic hearing during which she is encouraged to express her conflicts, fears and apprehensions.[14,28,61]

Effective management of the climacteric includes dispelling the fantasies and misconceptions a patient often has concerning the menopause—for instance, that it is usually accompanied by serious illness, and that it signifies the end of her sex life. An attempt should be made to assess whether the patient's appraisal of her own situation is realistic. When indicated, the physician can help her achieve more realistic attitudes, and encourage her to enjoy her new freedom from child rearing by extending her community activities, and reactivating dormant interests and ambitions. Since menopausal symptoms are often related to stress and disturbances in the home, the physician may also decide that counseling other family members is desirable for the patient's well-being.[8,11,28,30,55,68]

MANAGEMENT OF VAGINAL BLEEDING

During oral estrogen therapy, vaginal bleeding or blood-tinged staining in postmenopausal patients may result from benign endometrial proliferation or hyperplasia caused by the stimulating effect of excessive estrogen dosages.[59] However, bleeding in this age group is also frequently the first sign of endometrial or cervical carcinoma. It has been estimated that approximately one third of all cases of postmenopausal bleeding which are investigated by surgical curettage prove to be malignant in origin.[11] For this reason, most investigators emphasize the need for careful evaluation of any bleeding that develops during the course of estrogen therapy.

Bleeding or staining that appears within one week of stopping estrogen therapy—withdrawal bleeding—is recognized as a non-pathologic response to the cessation of estrogen stimulation of the endometrium. During the initial months of cyclic therapy in patients in their forties and fifties, it is not uncommon for withdrawal staining or moderate withdrawal bleeding to occur in the week when medication is stopped. Many clinicians regard this as a temporary and benign response. Simple withdrawal staining or bleeding usually ceases within a year after cyclic therapy has been initiated.[8,12,28,72]

If withdrawal bleeding is excessive or recurrent, or continues for more than ten days after cyclic estrogen therapy is interrupted, diagnostic curettage of the uterine cavity is usually considered essential. A cytologic finding of adenomatous hyperplasia is an indication for cautious observation and management of the patient. The condition may sometimes be reversed by adding progesterone at the end of several courses of cyclic estrogen therapy to induce medical curettage. Another cause of heavy withdrawal bleeding is activation of submucous leiomyomas which may be diagnosed during surgical curettage or by hysterography. In the presence of these fibroid tumors projecting into the uterine cavity, continued administration of estrogen is usually contraindicated.[11,72]

A second kind of bleeding or staining that may develop while estrogen therapy is being administered—breakthrough bleeding—is considered relatively more significant than withdrawal bleeding. Occasional breakthrough bleeding has been estimated to occur in twenty-five to thirty per cent of patients on continuous estrogen therapy. When it appears, many clinicians interrupt estrogen administration, and undertake a thorough diagnostic survey, which may include physical examination, curettage, and cervical biopsy. However, if the bleeding is moderate or represents a first episode, the patient may be closely observed for several weeks. If no pathology is found, and breakthrough bleeding stops within a short

40

time after cessation of therapy and does not reappear, estrogen replacement may be resumed at a lower dosage.[11,15,72]

Relief of climacteric symptoms can usually be achieved by giving estrogen in small, sub-bleeding doses. When larger doses are required to treat such specific symptoms as osteoporosis, or when a patient's endometrium is particularly susceptible to bleeding, controlled cyclic bleeding may be induced by the addition of progesterone at intervals during the estrogen therapy. The progestational agent is given for five to ten days, and planned bleeding can be expected to start within 48 to 72 hours after progesterone is withdrawn. A moderate flow of four or five days' duration results. Such regular shedding of the endometrium is considered to inhibit the development of adenomatous hyperplasia.[12,50,59,69]

MANAGEMENT OF SIDE EFFECTS

As with other medications, estrogen administration is capable of producing occasional side effects in susceptible patients. However, it has been noted that many of these symptoms abate or disappear with continued administration. Among phenomena observed are gastrointestinal disturbances, fluid retention and weight gain, breast and pelvic discomfort due to tissue engorgement, headache, vaginal discharge, and skin pigmentation.[8,12,15,58,72]

Clinicians have observed that these effects frequently result from oral estrogen dosages that are too high for an individual patient. Sensitivity has been shown to vary widely—some patients develop unwanted responses on relatively low doses, while others experience no adverse effects on quite high doses. In addition, the ability to tolerate the medication is often built up by starting with a small dosage, slowly increasing it, and persisting with this regimen for several months.[8,59]

The development of side effects in a given patient has been found to vary with the administration of different oral forms of estrogen. However, the natural conjugated estrogens have been cited by many investigators as being especially·well tolerated in most instances. [11,21,30,33,51,59,61,68,73,74]

V

Clinical Evidence of Therapeutic Benefits

BIOCHEMICAL STUDIES have only recently begun to elucidate the mechanisms by which estrogen produces its important metabolic and morphologic effects. The hormone appears to activate enzyme systems that play a key role in energy exchange within cells of such estrogen-sensitive tissues as the endometrium. It has also been found to aid protein synthesis by stimulating the formation of ribonucleic acid in uterine cells.[75]

Beneficial effects have been much more clearly defined on the clinical level. Reported results of estrogen replacement therapy in menopausal and postmenopausal patients indicate five major areas of clinical value.

PHYSICAL AND EMOTIONAL SYMPTOMS OF THE MENOPAUSAL SYNDROME

Numerous clinical investigations have shown that estrogen therapy dramatically alleviates many physical symptoms associated with the menopausal syndrome. In a series of two hundred private patients, ninety-eight per cent obtained lasting relief of hot flushes and ninety-five per cent were freed of distressing sweats.[23] Another study, on over one hundred patients, found relief in one hundred per cent of hot flushes, over three fourths of sweats, ninty per cent of headaches, and seventy-one per cent of arthralgias.[58]

Emotional symptoms that include depression and emotional instability, as well as what has been described as a "passive negativism" of personality, rank high among the troublesome manifestations of the menopausal syndrome.[20,69] A number of clinical investigators have noted the ability of estrogen therapy to counter these tendencies. Estrogen replacement was observed to produce "marked consistent improvement in mental health" in a group of four hundred and seventeen patients. Many had been severely disturbed and on the verge of seeking psychiatric intervention.[65]

Marked relief of emotional symptoms was also evident in a study of two hundred and eighty-eight patients, which excluded women with strong psychoneurotic tendencies. The investigator commented that "appetite increased, depression was supplanted by a sense of well-being, sleep improved, and a general improvement was noted in their outlook on life."[64] It has been pointed out that emotional symptoms may or may not be related to estrogen deficiency in a given person.[23] Common emotional symptoms, such as depression and insomnia, were relieved in about fifty per cent of a series of two hundred private patients treated with estrogen therapy.[23]

A relatively new focus of research is exploring the effects of estrogen therapy on senile mental involution. Several investigators have reported psychosocial benefits in studies undertaken to measure various responses to geriatric estrogen administration. Two thirds of fifty residents of a home for the aged evinced a greater interest in their environment and self-care, than prior to institution of estrogen treatment of their urogenital problems.[76]

44

VAGINAL TISSUES AND DYSPAREUNIA

Vaginal atrophy caused by postmenopausal estrogen deprivation may have several serious consequences. It can not only lead
to irritating vaginal discharge and infection, but also greatly reduce sexual satisfaction. Atrophic shrinking, thinning, and drying
of the vaginal mucosa often is asymptomatic except when intercourse is attempted. The resulting dyspareunia may cause feelings of guilt and sexual inadequacy in marital partners. It has been
noted that almost all postmenopausal patients who complain of
vaginal discharge admit to some discomfort during intercourse,
often sufficient to lead to abstinence.[26,69]

Experimental observation indicates that all phases of anatomic
and physiologic response to sexual stimulation are reduced in
women of advanced years. Production of vaginal lubrication is
delayed, and the vagina loses much of its ability to expand volun-
tarily during sexual tension. Orgasm is generally shortened in
duration, and may also be accompanied by painful uterine contractions.[26]

Numerous investigators have described the dramatic reversal of
vaginal atrophy produced by estrogen therapy. In the words of
one, the postmenopausal vagina "responds phenomenally in the
form of epithelial growth to the administration of estrogen. The
number of epithelial layers increases from approximately six to
thirty. There is an increase in the glycogen content of the epithelial
cells, favoring the formation of lactic acid and the return of the
normal flora. Cornification and shedding of the superficial layers
of epithelium help rid the vagina of invading organisms." [11](Fig. 6.)

A typical result of estrogen therapy was the relief of the vaginal
irritation and dyspareunia due to atrophic vaginitis in all of the
affected patients in a study of two hundred menopausal and postmenopausal cases.[23] Another investigation reports that adequate

45

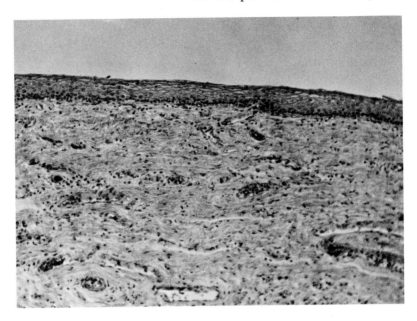

FIG. 6a   Biopsy of vaginal mucosa of postmenopausal woman before estrogen treatment; note thin layer of epithelial cells and moderate submucosal leukocytic infiltration.

estrogen replacement therapy corrects involutional changes in the genital tract and thereby promotes the return of physical capacity for sexual performance. It is further noted that combined estrogen and progesterone, supplied continuously, often relieved the cramp-like pain of uterine contractions suffered by some older women during orgasm.[26]

URINARY STRUCTURES AND PELVIC SUPPORT

Atrophic changes resulting from estrogen deficiency may extend beyond the vagina and involve adjacent urinary structures

46

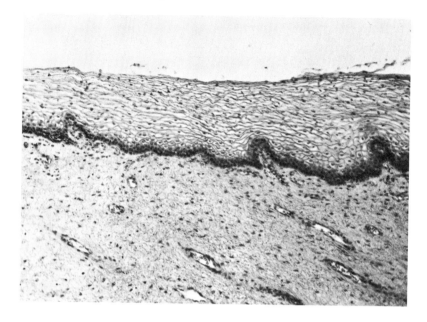

FIG. 6b Biopsy of same vagina after treatment with estrogen; note numerous well-differentiated epithelial cells and absence of leukocytic infiltration of submucosa.

and the muscles and ligaments that support the uterus and other pelvic organs. When the deficiency persists for many years, postmenopausal patients often develop such distressing conditions as dysuria, urinary frequency, or incontinence, as well as uterine prolapse, cystocele, and rectocele. Increasing clinical evidence suggests that these conditions may be largely prevented or reversed with estrogen therapy.[14,31,77-79]

Urinary problems arise from involution, inflammation, or decreased tone occurring in the tissues surrounding the urethral meatus, the urethra itself, the trigone area of the bladder, or the bladder's muscular wall. All these structures have been found to respond to the influence of estrogen.[28,31,78,79]

Beneficial results were observed when estrogen was adminis-

47

tered to a series of twenty-nine elderly, institutionalized women with chronic, severe genitourinary symptoms. Before treatment, all had suffered from atrophic vaginitis, and most had exhibited a strong odor of urine indicating incontinence. Many were found to have some degree of prolapse, cystocele, and rectocele. After three months of estrogen replacement therapy, objective improvement was noted in every patient. In two cases, partial prolapse was relieved; cystoceles and urethroceles appeared to be less prominent.[76]

Relaxation of the ligaments that support the uterus, and of the muscles of the pelvic floor, is believed responsible for external protrusion of the uterus, rectum, or bladder. A number of investigators have observed that estrogen therapy helps restore tone to pelvic supporting structures, and may even obviate the need for surgery in some patients.[65,73,77]

Estrogen therapy has also been found to be of value before and after essential reconstructive surgery is performed on the vagina and pelvic floor. The treated tissues are noted to be in better condition for surgery, and subsequent healing is promoted.[78,80]

BONE METABOLISM AND OSTEOPOROSIS

Osteoporotic loss of bone density occurs in about twenty-five per cent of postmenopausal women.[33,40,43,70] Although the specific mechanism is still unresolved, estrogen deficiency appears to be a very important factor in the development of osteoporosis. New technics for detecting small degrees of bone loss indicate that the process begins soon after menopause.[32,34,43]

No evidence has been found that therapy can restore bone that has already been lost. However, three long term studies have established the effectiveness of estrogen replacement in preventing, or at least retarding, postmenopausal osteoporosis. Further height loss due to vertebral compression fractures was halted, or markedly reduced, in twenty of twenty-two patients who were given estrogen therapy after clinical effects of osteoporosis—including loss of as much as five inches of stature—had been observed. The same study showed that twenty-seven patients who were treated with estrogen for reasons unrelated to bone loss remained free of significant back pain, height loss, or vertebral compression during four to twenty-five years of replacement therapy.[37]

During a study involving twelve hundred patient-years of estrogen administration to two hundred and twenty women with postmenopausal osteoporosis, no further fractures or loss of height were observed, even though both symptoms had been prominent features of the patients' condition prior to treatment.[35] When a sensitive method of detecting osteoporosis was used in one hundred and forty-nine postmenopausal women, eighty-seven of whom received estrogen therapy, it was observed that treated patients lost less bone than did untreated patients. The investigator concluded that hormone supplementation either prevented osteoporosis, or delayed it for at least 10 years.[32]

BLOOD LIPIDS
AND ATHEROSCLEROSIS

Epidemiologic evidence suggests that endogenous estrogen production plays a role in conferring resistance to atherosclerosis during the premenopausal years, and laboratory data indicate that estrogens influence blood-lipid levels in experimental animals.[44] Definitive evidence on the question whether estrogen replacement therapy can extend protection against other manifestations of atherosclerosis in postmenopausal women awaits completion of long term clinical studies which are in progress.

49

However, a few studies on human subjects have already yielded preliminary results. Several have been carried out on women who underwent premature menopause as a result of surgical removal of the ovaries. One hundred and two such castrated patients were compared with one hundred and twelve women of similar age who had undergone only hysterectomy. After an average interval of ten years postsurgery, nineteen of the castrates were found to have experienced such cardiovascular disorders as angina, coronary infarct, or peripheral vascular disease, compared to five of the hysterectomized patients. And in a follow-up two years later, seven additional cardiovascular events were found to have occurred in the castrated group in contrast to none among the controls. Furthermore, a small group of castrates treated with estrogen experienced a rate of cardiovascular complications almost as low as that of the uncastrated controls.[46,81] A similar study comparing the cardiovascular status of castrated patients who were being given estrogen therapy with untreated castrated patients found that the treated patients experienced a lower incidence of hypertension and fewer abnormal electrocardiograms.[48]

Although prevention of atherosclerosis has not yet been demonstrated in women who have experienced spontaneous menopause, administration of estrogen has been shown to shift their serum lipid patterns toward those seen in premenopausal women. A number of investigators have reported that estrogen therapy lowers postmenopausal serum cholesterol, increases alpha lipoprotein, and lowers the cholesterol-phospholipid ratio—changes currently thought to be desirable in the primary and secondary prevention of atherosclerosis.[44,48,82]

VI

Evidence Regarding Carcinogenesis

PERIODIC DISCUSSIONS of a possible relationship between estrogen therapy and cancer of the reproductive organs have stemmed largely from indirect evidence reported in an earlier period. It was observed, for example, that ovariectomy sometimes ameliorated the clinical course of breast cancer in humans.[83] More recently it was found that administration of estrogen to certain highly selected, inbred strains of mice was followed by a high incidence of breast cancer.[84] It was also noted that estrogen is chemically related to such carcinogens as methylcholanthrene.[85,86] Additionally, a high incidence of endometrial cancer was reported by some investigators in postmenopausal patients with feminizing ovarian tumors that secreted estrogen.[87]

Numerous modern investigations have better clarified the factors involved in the proliferation of reproductive tissues and the effects of estrogen on the growth of malignant tumors of the breasts and genital structures. While a few investigators[86,88] feel that the evidence concerning a causal relationship between estrogen and cancer is still inconclusive, most, including specialists, appear to conclude that there is little convincing evidence that estrogen plays a causative role in the induction of cancer.[11,12,15,19,30] [33,58,61,66,75,89-92] This viewpoint emerges from the findings of four different kinds of studies.

ANIMAL FINDINGS

The classic induction of breast cancer in mice appears to be a special situation, since two other factors are invariably present in addition to estrogen administration. The inbred mice are of a genetic strain that shows a high spontaneous incidence of breast cancer even when not so treated. Furthermore, they carry a virus-like tumor agent which is transferred through the mother's milk. Neither factor has been demonstrated to operate in the human.[93] Moreover, calculations indicate that in a 20 year period it would be impossible to administer to women estrogen doses equivalent to those used to induce cancer in the mice studies.[92,94]

Although estrogen has been associated with an increased incidence of breast and genital cancer in some rat and rabbit experiments,[86] it has consistently failed to do so in long term studies in monkeys.[93] Reporting on one such experiment, the investigators stated, "As far as we are able to determine, the colony of 21 monkeys forming the basis of this report received the largest total dosage of estrogens ever administered to living animals, and in spite of this no neoplasms were produced." Periodic biopsies of breast and endometrial tissues were studied microscopically. Three of the monkeys were given intramuscular injections and pellet implants for over seven years and were not autopsied until 14 years after initiation of treatment.[95]

While animal experiments are not necessarily predictive for humans, it has been noted that closer correlations in results can generally be expected when the animal is more closely related to man.[93] The mouse experiments, which have been called misleading, resulted in an undue emphasis being placed on the chemical similarity between estrogens and some carcinogenic substances.[11,50]

PHYSIOLOGIC OBSERVATIONS

Cancer of the reproductive organs in women occurs more often when estrogen levels are low rather than high. The vast majority of uterine cancers develop in women after age 40, when endogenous estrogen production is declining. The incidence of breast cancer also increases with age. Moreover, development of breast cancer during pregnancy is rare, and estrogen production is higher at this time than in any other period of life.[69,94] It is infrequent even in women who have had many children in rapid succession and been exposed to almost continuous high concentrations of estrogen.

Studies that have linked the development of uterine cancer with the adenomatous hyperplasia that sometimes develops during estrogen therapy have been challenged statistically, and so have observations that estrogen-producing ovarian tumors increase the incidence of uterine cancer. Neither of these contentions is considered to be physiologic proof of a causal relationship between estrogen administration and cancer.[11,30,61,89,94,96-98]

One investigator has concluded, "Although it is theoretically possible that the administration of estrogen during the *preclinical* stage of malignancy of the generative organs could hasten the appearance of its signs and symptoms, the eventual progress of the disease cannot be arrested by withholding estrogen."[11]

EPIDEMIOLOGIC DATA

Included in the evidence against estrogen carcinogenesis is the absence of a detectable increase in the incidence of female reproductive cancers since the therapeutic use of estrogen began in the early 1930's. Mortality rates for uterine and breast cancer in the years 1930, 1940, and 1950 were compared.[99] They turned out not to differ significantly for any age group, despite the steadily increasing application of estrogen therapy. A study covering the years 1930 to 1956 found that there had been no rise in the mortality rate from breast cancer, and a slight decline in the rate from uterine cancer.[100] A summary of data on the incidence of and mortality from breast cancer in Connecticut between 1941 and 1954, and in New York State between 1942 and 1953, found that although the rates fluctuated slightly, there was no consistent or significant upward trend.[90] Similarly, the breast cancer mortality rate in Massachusetts has not been observed to increase materially over the past thirty years.[55]

CLINICAL STUDIES

Occasional cases of breast or uterine cancer have been reported in patients who had previously or simultaneously been treated with estrogen for various conditions.[86,89,93] However, the overwhelming majority of investigations reveal rates below those that could have been anticipated on statistical grounds for this age group.

For example, only twenty-three cases of uterine cancer were observed in patients who received estrogen therapy during a 20 year period at the Sloan Hospital for Women in New York.[101]

The results of five major studies[19,31,37,40,50,102] of long term therapeutic administration of estrogen have been totaled. Statistical

54

projections from known rates suggested that ninety-six cases of cancer of the breast and uterus could be expected to develop among the combined total of 1,422 treated patients. Instead, only five uterine cancers were observed (no cases involved the breast); all occurred during a study of the effects of estrogen therapy on the development of postmenopausal osteoporosis.[37] Four of the five observed uterine cancers were endometrial and developed during the first 15 years of the 25 year study, when estrogen therapy had been applied continuously. After the adoption of a cyclic regimen in 1948, only one cervical cancer *in situ* was seen, and no invasive endometrial or breast cancers developed.[33,103]

An absence of malignancies has been a consistent finding of many long term clinical studies. No cancers appeared in osteoporotic patients treated cyclically with estrogen for a total of 1,100 patient-years, although the investigator had expected five or six cases in view of the recorded incidence of cancer in women of the comparable postmenopausal age group.[40] Additionally, in a group of three hundred and four women treated with estrogen for up to 27 years (average: 7.8 years), with a breast exposure of 2,387 patient-years and a genital exposure of 1,852 patient-years, eighteen cases of reproductive cancer were anticipated statistically, but no malignancies occurred.[89]

VII

Classification of Estrogens and Important Clinical Characteristics

GENERAL CLASSIFICATION

In general, estrogens fall into three categories: naturally occurring, nonsteroidal, and chemically modified.

NATURALLY OCCURRING ESTROGENS are steroid hormones, their basic nucleus consisting of the cyclopentano-phenanthrene or steroid ring system. They occur either as conjugates or as free estrogens.

Conjugated estrogens: Biochemically speaking, conjugation is the chemical linkage by a natural process of two compounds in the living body. In pregnancy, estrogens are excreted mostly as water-soluble conjugates: as sulfates in pregnant mares, *e.g.,* estrone sulfate, equilin sulfate, etc.; as glucuronides in pregnant women, *e.g.,* estriol glucuronide. (The urine of pregnant mares is the richer and more potent source of natural estrogens.)

In nature, the conjugated estrogens exist mostly in the form of their corresponding sodium salts.

56

Estrogens can be linked to a chemical radical in the laboratory, but those manufactured in this way are not designated as conjugated estrogens. For example, 17β-estradiol benzoate, prepared in the laboratory from 17β-estradiol and benzoic acid, is known as an esterified estrogen.

In other words, the term "conjugated estrogens" applies only to those estrogen derivatives that occur naturally in the living body, and not to those synthesized in the laboratory.

Natural (conjugated)

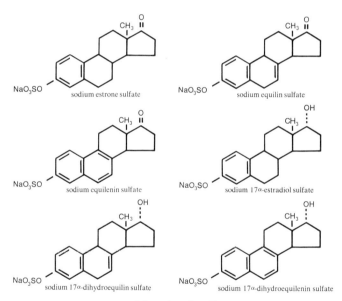

sodium estrone sulfate

sodium equilin sulfate

sodium equilenin sulfate

sodium 17α-estradiol sulfate

sodium 17α-dihydroequilin sulfate

sodium 17α-dihydroequilenin sulfate

and other conjugated steroids

Free estrogens: These are estrogens that have been released by hydrolysis from naturally occurring conjugation, *e.g.,* estrone, estriol, 17β-estradiol, etc. (Because of the difficulty in concentrating and purifying the conjugated water-soluble forms of estrogens, the water-insoluble free forms were the first to be presented for therapeutic use.)

Natural (free)

estrone

NONSTEROIDAL ESTROGENS are body-foreign substances with estrogen-like activity. Their formulas are totally unlike that of natural estrogens. Coal tar derivatives such as the stilbenes are typical.

diethylstilbestrol

Other nonsteroidal estrogens are: benzestrol, chlorotrianisene, dienestrol, diethylstilbestrol dipropionate, hexestrol, mestilbol, methallenestril, and promethestrol dipropionate.

58

CHEMICALLY MODIFIED ESTROGENS have been synthesized in the laboratory from natural estrogens but have no counterpart in nature; hence they are body-foreign substances.

17β-estradiol benzoate   ethynyl estradiol

Other semisynthetic estrogens are: mestranol (the 3-methyl ether of ethynyl estradiol), 17β-estradiol dipropionate, and piperazine estrone sulfate.

CLINICAL CHARACTERISTICS

Natural (conjugated) estrogens are highly potent when given orally. In addition, they are well tolerated, and comparatively free from side effects.

In their conjugated form, estrogens are water-soluble and orally active to a much greater degree than the corresponding free forms of estrogen. There is considerable evidence that conjugated estrogens are not so readily destroyed by the liver as the free estrogens, and that this accounts for the greater activity when taken by mouth.

Natural (free) estrogens are oil-soluble and therefore active parenterally. When given orally, however, they are relatively weak, resulting in metabolic waste of active material.

Some *nonsteroidal* and *chemically modified estrogens* are orally active, but accompanied by more side effects in a substantial percentage of cases.

Bibliography

1   Talbot, N. B.: Adolescence, in Holt, L. E., Jr., McIntosh, R., and Barnett, H. L.: Pediatrics, ed. 13, New York, Appleton-Century-Crofts Inc., 1962, p. 19.
2   Rogers, J.: Endocrine and Metabolic Aspects of Gynecology, Philadelphia, W. B. Saunders Company, 1963, pp. 1, 101, 118.
3   Lloyd, G. W.: The Ovaries, in Williams, R. H.: Textbook of Endocrinology, ed. 4, Philadelphia, W. B. Saunders Company, 1968, pp. 459, 513.
4   Van Wyk, J. J., and Grumbach, M. M.: Disorders of Sex Differentiation, in Williams, R. H.: Textbook of Endocrinology, ed. 4, Philadelphia, W. B. Saunders Company, 1968, p. 537.
5   Daughaday, W. H.: The Adenohypophysis, in Williams, R. H.: Textbook of Endocrinology, ed. 4, Philadelphia, W. B. Saunders Company, 1968, pp. 27, 39.
6   Reichlin, S.: Neuroendocrinology, in Williams, R. H.: Textbook of Endocrinology, ed. 4, Philadelphia, W. B. Saunders Company, 1968, pp. 967, 975, 985, 1011.
7   Stevens, V. C., and Vorys, N.: Gonadotropin Secretion in the Normal Cycle, in Greenblatt, R. B.: Ovulation, Philadelphia, J. B. Lippincott Company, 1966, p. 16.
8   Paschkis, K. E., Rakoff, A. E., Cantarow, A., and Rupp, J. J.: Clinical Endocrinology, ed. 3, New York, Hoeber Medical Division, Harper & Row, Publishers, 1967, pp. 521, 588, 600, 656.
9   Riley, G. M.: Endocrinology of the climacteric, Clin. Obstet. Gynec. 7:432 (June) 1964.
10 MacGregor, T. N.: The endocrinology of the menopause, Practitioner 182:539 (May) 1959.
11 Israel, S. L.: Diagnosis and Treatment of Menstrual Disorders and Sterility, New York, Hoeber Medical Division, Harper & Row, Publishers, 1967, pp. 32, 390.
12 Greenblatt, R. B.: Estrogen therapy for postmenopausal females, New Eng. J. Med. 272:305 (Feb. 11) 1965.

61

13 Overstreet, E. W.: Endocrine management of the geriatric woman, Amer. J. Obstet. Gynec. *95*:354 (June 1) 1966.

14 Beecham, C. T., and Forman, I.: The Menopause and the Climacteric, in Willson, J. R., Beecham, C. T., and Carrington, E. R.: Obstetrics and Gynecology, ed. 2, St. Louis, The C. V. Mosby Company, 1963, p. 671.

15 Kupperman, H. S.: The menopausal woman and sex hormones, Med. Aspects Hum. Sexuality *1*:64 (Sept.) 1967.

16 McCandless, F. D.: Emotional problems of the climacteric, Clin. Obstet. Gynec. *7*:489 (June) 1964.

17 Kupperman, H. S.: Human Endocrinology, Philadelphia, F. A. Davis Company, 1963, vol. 2, p. 426.

18 Neugarten, B.L., and Kraines, R. J.: "Menopausal symptoms" in women of various ages, Psychosom. Med. *27*:266 (May-June) 1965.

19 Bakke, J. L.: A teaching device to assist active therapeutic intervention in the menopause, Western J. Surg. Obstet. Gynec. *71*:241 (Nov.-Dec.) 1963.

20 Malleson, J.: Climacteric stress: its empirical management, Brit. Med. J. *2*:1422 (Dec. 15) 1956.

21 Sturgis, S. H.: Treatment of ovarian insufficiency, Amer. J. Nurs. *64*:113 (Jan.) 1964.

22 O'Neill, D.: Psychiatric disturbances of the menopause, Practitioner *182*:565 (May) 1959.

23 Kaufman, S. A.: Limited relationship of maturation index to estrogen therapy for menopausal symptoms, Obstet. Gynec. *30*:399 (Sept.) 1967.

24 Lang, W. R., and Aponte, G. E.: Gross and microscopic anatomy of the aged female reproductive organs, Clin. Obstet. Gynec. *10*: 454 (Sept.) 1967.

25 Kretzschmar, W. A., and Stoddard, F. J.: Physiologic changes in the aging female, Clin. Obstet. Gynec. *7*:451 (June) 1964.

26 Masters, W. H., and Johnson, V. E.: Human Sexual Response, Boston, Little, Brown and Company, 1966, p. 223.

27 Pratt, J. P.: Gynecologic problems of aging, Postgrad. Med. *37*:213 (Feb.) 1965.

28 Pearl, M. J., and Plotz, E. J.: Management of the climacteric patient, Clin. Obstet. Gynec. *7*:476 (June) 1964.

29 Williams, D. I.: The skin and the menopause, Practitioner *182*:574 (May) 1959.

30 Rogers, J.: Hormonal therapy in the menopause, J. St. Barnabas Med. Center *1*:83 (Mar.) 1962.

31 Schleyer-Saunders, E.: The management of the menopause, Med. Press *244*:337 (Oct. 19) 1960.

32 Davis, M. E., Strandjord, N. M., and Lanzl, L. H.: Estrogens and the aging process—The detection, prevention, and retardation of osteoporosis, J.A.M.A. *196*:129 (Apr. 18) 1966.

Bibliography

33 Henneman, P. H.: Postmenopausal osteoporosis, Clin. Obstet. Gynec. 7:531 (June) 1964.

34 Meema, H. E., Bunker, M. L., and Meema, S.: Loss of compact bone due to menopause, Obstet. Gynec. 26:333 (Sept.) 1965.

35 Gordan, G. S., and Eisenberg, E.: The effect of oestrogens, androgens and corticoids on skeletal kinetics in man, Proc. Roy. Soc. Med. 56:1027 (Nov.) 1963.

36 Jasani, C., Nordin, B. E. C., Smith, D. A., and Swanson, I.: Spinal osteoporosis and the menopause, Proc. Roy. Soc. Med. 58:441 (June) 1965.

37 Wallach, S., and Henneman, P. H.: Prolonged estrogen therapy in postmenopausal women, J.A.M.A. 171:1637 (Nov. 21) 1959.

38 Dent, C. E., and Watson, L.: Osteoporosis, Postgrad. Med. J. 42: (Suppl.) 583 (Oct.) 1966.

39 Urist, M. R.: Osteoporosis, Ann. Rev. Med. 13:273, 1962.

40 Gordan, G. S.: Osteoporosis diagnosis and treatment, Texas Med. 57:740 (Sept.) 1961.

41 Nordin, B.E.C.: The pathogenesis of osteoporosis, Lancet 1:1011 (May 13) 1961.

42 Young, M. M., and Nordin, B. E. C.: Effects of natural and artificial menopause on plasma and urinary calcium and phosphorus, Lancet 2:118 (July 15) 1967.

43 Selle, W. A., and Jurist, J. M.: The onset of postmenopausal osteoporosis as studied by a new technique, J. Amer. Geriat. Soc. 14: 930 (Sept.) 1966.

44 Berkson, D. M., Stamler, J., and Cohen, D. B.: Ovarian function and coronary atherosclerosis, Clin. Obstet. Gynec. 7:504 (June) 1964.

45 Parrish, H. M., Carr, C. A., Hall, D. G., and King, T. M.: Time interval from castration in premenopausal women to development of excessive coronary atherosclerosis, Amer. J. Obstet. Gynec. 99:155 (Sept. 15) 1967.

46 Higano, N., Robinson, R. W., and Cohen, W. D.: Increased incidence of cardiovascular disease in castrated women, New Eng. J. Med. 268:1123 (May 16) 1963.

47 Oliver, M. F., and Boyd, G. S.: Effect of bilateral ovariectomy on coronary-artery disease and serum-lipid levels, Lancet 2:690 (Oct. 31) 1959.

48 Davis, M. E., Jones, R. J., and Jarolim, C.: Long-term estrogen substitution and atherosclerosis, Amer. J. Obstet. Gynec. 82:1003 (Nov.) 1961.

49 Morton, J. H.: Menopause, in Conn, H. F.: Current Therapy 1967, Philadelphia, W. B. Saunders Company, 1967, p. 724.

50 Wilson, R. A., Brevetti, R. E., and Wilson, T. A.: Specific procedures for the elimination of the menopause, Western J. Surg. Obstet. Gynec. 71:110 (May-June) 1963.

51 Lin, T.-J., and Lin, S.-C.: The vaginal cytogram, J.A.M.A. *185*:844 (Sept. 14) 1963.

52 Hammond, D. O.: Endocrine vaginal cytology, GP *30*:123 (Sept.) 1964.

53 Masukawa, T.: Vaginal smears in women past 40 years of age, with emphasis on their remaining hormonal activity, Obstet. Gynec. *16*:407 (Oct.) 1960.

54 Liu, W.: Letters—Continuous estrogen treatment in women, J.A.M.A. *192*:332 (Apr. 26) 1965.

55 Goldfarb, A. F.: Menopause—The climacteric: Its role in aging, Med. Sci. *18*:48 (Feb.) 1967.

56 Christian, C. D.: Current Concepts of Estrogen Replacement Therapy —Transcript of a Round Table Conference, Excerpta Medica Foundation, 1966.

57 Wilson, R. A., and Wilson, T. A.: The fate of the nontreated postmenopausal woman: A plea for the maintenance of adequate estrogen from puberty to the grave, J. Amer. Geriat. Soc. *11*:347 (Apr.) 1963.

58 Rhoades, F. P.: Minimizing the menopause, J. Amer. Geriat. Soc. *15*:346 (Apr.) 1967.

59 Parks, J.: Care of the postmenopausal patient, Postgrad. Med. *42*:275 (Oct.) 1967.

60 McGoogan, L. S.: Treatment of the menopause, S. Dakota J. Med. *18*:17 (June) 1965.

61 Hunt, W., and Beecham, C. T.: Current concepts of estrogen-replacement therapy, Bull. Geisinger Med. Center *18*:119 (Nov.) 1966.

62 Francis, W. G.: Long-term estrogen and progestin therapy, Appl. Ther. *9*:833 (Oct.) 1967.

63 Barnes, A. C.: Is menopause a disease?, Consultant *2*:22 (June) 1962.

64 Tramont, C. B.: Cyclic hormone therapy—A report on 305 cases, Geriatrics *21*:212 (Nov.) 1966.

65 Meyer, H.: Maturation index and cyclic hormone therapy (limitation of the aging process), Nebraska Med. J. *52*:65 (Feb.) 1967.

66 McEwen, D. C.: Estrogen replacement therapy at menopause, Canad. Nurse *63*:34 (Feb.) 1967.

67 Davis, M. E.: Modern management of menopausal patient, Curr. Med. Digest *33*:39 (Jan.) 1966.

68 Lammert, A. C.: The menopause—a physiologic process, Amer. J. Nurs. *62*:56 (Feb.) 1962.

69 Cameron, W. J.: Endocrine therapy in the menopause, GP *33*:110 (May) 1966.

70 Dunn, A. W.: Senile osteoporosis, Geriatrics *22*:175 (Nov.) 1967.

71 Chu, L. S. W., and Abramson, D. I.: Diagnosis and treatment of osteoporosis, Geriatrics *18*:679 (Sept.) 1963.

72 Kistner, R. W.: Feminine forever? An evaluation of therapy during perimenopause, Med. Sci. *18*:42 (Oct.) 1967.

73 McEwen, D. C.: Ovarian failure and the menopause, Canad. Med. Ass. J. *92*:962 (May 1) 1965.

74 Johnson, C. G.: Hormonal therapy in obstetrics and gynecology, Memphis Mid-South Med. J. *40*:267 (Aug.) 1965.

75 Taymor, M. L.: Advances in endocrinology: A ten year review, Clin. Obstet. Gynec. *10*: 667 (Sept.) 1967.

76 Siegel, I., Zelinger, B. B., and Kanter, A. E.: Estrogen therapy for urogenital conditions in the aged, Amer. J. Obstet. Gynec. *84*: 505 (Aug. 15) 1962.

77 Anderson, H. E.: Clinical use of estrogen in uterine prolapse, J.A.M.A. *168*:173 (Sept. 13) 1958.

78 Hamblen, E. C.: The use of estrogens in obstetrics and gynecology, Clin. Obstet. Gynec. *3*:1021 (Dec.) 1960.

79 Youssef, A. F.: Drug effect on the female bladder and its sphincter mechanism, Obstet. Gynec. *13*:61 (Jan.) 1959.

80 Arnas, G. M., and Long, J. P.: Pelvic relaxation in the elderly female, Clin. Obstet. Gynec. *10*:488 (Sept.) 1967.

81 Robinson, R. W., Higano, N., and Cohen, W. D.: Increased incidence of coronary heart disease in women castrated prior to menopause, Arch. Intern. Med. *104*:908 (Dec.) 1959.

82 Marmorston, J., Magidson, O., Lewis, J. J., Mehl, J., Moore, F. J., and Bernstein, J.: Effect of small doses of estrogen on serum lipids in female patients with myocardial infarction, New Eng. J. Med. *258*:583 (Mar.) 1958.

83 Beatson, G. T.: On the treatment of inoperable cases of carcinoma of the mamma: Suggestions for a new method of treatment, with illustrative cases, Lancet *2*:104 (July 11) 1896.

84 Lacassagne, A.: Apparition de cancers de la mammelle chez la souris mâle soumise à des injections de folliculine, C.R. Acad. Sc.*195*: 630 (Oct.) 1932.

85 Dodds, E. C.: Synthetic oestrogens, Brit. Med. Bull. *11*:131 (May) 1955.

86 Hertz, R.: The role of steroid hormones in the etiology and pathogenesis of cancer, Amer. J. Obstet. Gynec. *98*:1013 (Aug. 1) 1967.

87 Greene, J. W., Jr.: Feminizing mesenchymomas (granulosa-cell and theca-cell tumors) with associated endometrial carcinoma, Amer. J. Obstet. Gynec. *74*:31 (July) 1957.

88 Novak, E. R.: Replacement therapy of the menopause, Johns Hopkins Med. J. *120*:408 (June) 1967.

89 Wilson, R. A.: The roles of estrogen and progesterone in breast and genital cancer, J.A.M.A. *182*:327 (Oct. 27) 1962.

90 Shimkin, M. B.: Cancer of the breast—Some old facts and new prospectives, J.A.M.A. *183*:358 (Feb. 2) 1963.

91 Davis, M. E.: Long-term estrogen substitution after the menopause Clin. Obstet. Gynec. *7*:558 (June) 1964.

92 Leis, H. P., Jr.: Endocrine prophylaxis of breast cancer with cyclic estrogen and progesterone, Int. Surg. 45:496 (May) 1966.

93 Drill, V. A.: Relationship of administered estrogen, progesterone, and oral contraceptives to cancer of breast and genital organs of women, Pacif. Med. Surg. 73:395 (Nov.-Dec.) 1965.

94 Wilson, R.A.: The estrogen cancer myth, Clin. Med. 71:1343 (Aug.) 1964.

95 Geschickter, C. F., and Hartman, C. G.: Mammary response to prolonged estrogenic stimulation in the monkey, Cancer 12:767 (July-Aug.) 1959.

96 Roddick, J. W., Jr., and Greene, R.R.: Relation of ovarian stromal hyperplasia to endometrial carcinoma, Amer. J. Obstet. Gynec. 73:843 (Apr.) 1957.

97 Boss, J. H., Scully, R. E., Wegner, K. H., and Cohen, R. B.: Structural variations in the adult ovary—Clinical significance, Obstet. Gynec. 25:747 (June) 1965.

98 Larson, J. A.: Estrogens and endometrial carcinoma, Obstet. Gynec. 3:551 (May) 1954.

99 Shelton, E. K.: The pros and cons of estrogen administration after the menopause, J. Amer. Geriat. Soc. 4:348 (Apr.) 1956.

100 Hammond, E. C.: Trends in cancer death rates and cure rates, Ann. Intern. Med. 50:300 (Feb.) 1959.

101 Gusberg, S. B., and Hall, R. E.: Precursors of corpus cancer. III. The appearance of cancer of the endometrium in estrogenically conditioned patients, Obstet. Gynec. 17:397 (Apr.) 1961.

102 Geist, S. H., and Salmon, U. J.: Are estrogens carcinogenic in the human female? The effect of long-continued estrogen administration upon the uterine and vaginal mucosa of the human female, Amer. J. Obstet. Gynec. 41:29 (Jan.) 1941.

103 Geller, W.: Treatment of menopausal problems—relationship between estrogen therapy and cancer, Mod. Treatm. 5:564 (May) 1968.

Revised October, 1968
A 8741-50-1168

NOTES

NOTES

NOTES

NOTES

NOTES

NOTES